"To my wife who brought color to my life"

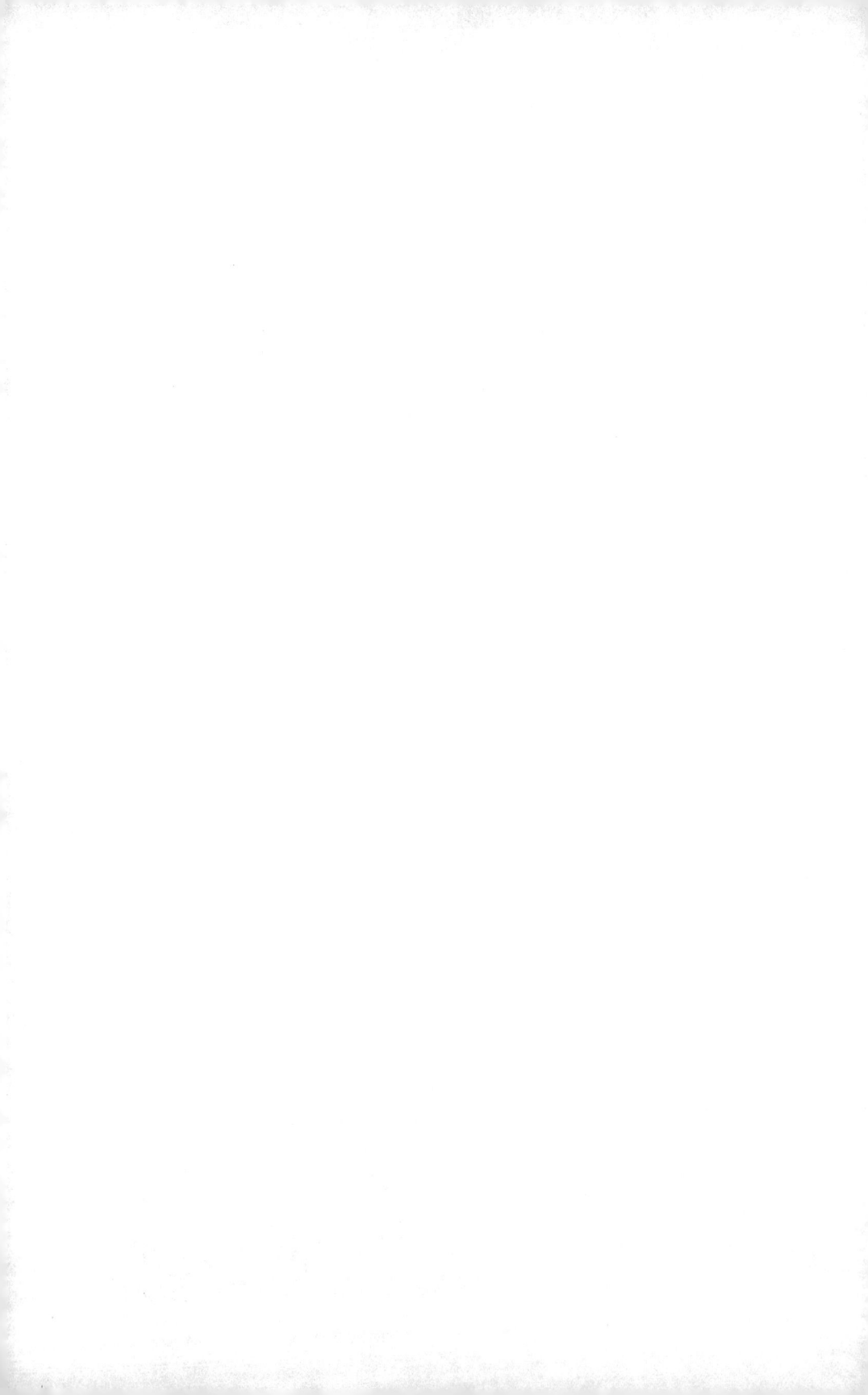

CONTENTS

Chapter 1	1
What is Hypnosis?	2
Chapter 2	6
What is Hypnosis Good For?	7
Chapter 3	12
How to Induce Hypnosis?	13
Chapter 4	21
How to deepen Hypnosis?	22
Chapter 5	26
How to implement the treatment approach?	27
Chapter 6	30
How to terminate Hypnosis?	31
Chapter 7	34
Hypnotic Phenomena	35
Chapter 8	42
Cautions, Contraindication and Resistance	43
Chapter 9	47
Self Hypnosis	48
Chapter 10	50
Conversational hypnosis	51
Chapter 11	54

How to educate your clients?	55
Chapter 12	57
Hypnosis for compassion fatigue	58

CHAPTER 1

WHAT IS HYPNOSIS?

Welcome to the book, "Hypnosis: A First Look".

Let's start with the definition of hypnosis. As Forbes Robbins Blair mentions in his book, "Instant Self-Hypnosis", The truth is that there is no consensus about the definition of hypnosis. For the sake of simplicity, we use the definition of American Society of Clinical Hypnosis in this book: "Hypnosis is a phenomenon that is characterized by a state of attentive, receptive concentration, containing three concurrent features of varying degrees: Dissociation, Absorption, and Suggestion." All three of these need to be present for hypnosis to occur.

The history of hypnosis dates to the Egyptians' sleep temples 4000 years ago. The concept of modern hypnosis has evolved a lot, since being introduced by the German physician, Franz Mesmer. Even though our understanding of hypnosis is totally different from that of Mesmer's, we can call him the father of modern hypnosis.

Most of the time hypnosis is done with closed eyes and in a relaxed position, but it can happen with open eyes while the subject is involved in a physical activity. For example, a soccer goalkeeper can be in a state of hypnosis during the game.

People experience hypnosis differently, so it's very hard to say if it's an altered state of mind or not. The mechanism of hypnosis has been the source of controversy for years. The one mechanism that I resonated with the best is called the Meta-Cognition Game. However, I should confess that this model is more descriptive than explanatory. By definition, meta-cognition is an awareness and understanding of one's own thought processes. In other words, a meta-cognition is a cognition about cognition.

Theoretical models of hypnosis are beyond the scope of this book. In this book, we will focus on the practical aspects of hypnosis. The bottom line is that hypnosis often helps us to change the physiology of the body, as well as our perceptions and behaviors. Symptom therapy like pain relief techniques is a good example. Hypnosis is also a great tool to tap into the unconscious mind of the subject and as a result of that, it can be used as a vehicle for other approaches like psychotherapy.

People differ in their amount of responsiveness to hypnosis. The degree of this responsiveness is called *hypnotizability*. As a rule of thumb, 15% of everyone in a given population is highly hypnotizable and 5% is not hypnotizable at all. It looks like the degree of hypnotizability does not change over time. So, meditation or other similar exercises have no effect on hypnotizability. However, some psychological conditions like depression can mask hypnotisability. A highly hypnotizable depressed patient may lose the ability to be hypnotized. But he or she will be hypnotizable again two weeks after starting antidepressant medication.

For medical purposes, light to medium hypnosis is enough. The subject does not need to be highly hypnotizable to benefit from hypnosis.

When it comes to hypnosis, this question is often asked, "What are the differences and similarities between hypnosis and meditation?" As mentioned earlier, the goal of this book is not to focus on theory. However, as a short answer, it looks like they are both a metacognition game; but in different directions. In hypnosis, you create new cognitions, while in meditation you try to get rid of the made-up cognitions. It's like a "two-way" road. In hypnosis, you travel in one direction but in meditation, you travel in the opposite direction. At the end of the day, it's the same road: a metacognition game.

Every hypnosis is self-hypnosis. In other words, the whole process is about the native talent of the subject and not the power of the hypnotherapist or hypnotist. For sure, the hypnotist should be well trained but at the end of the day, it's a skill everybody can learn and practice.

From the therapeutic perspective, it is important to understand that hypnosis is like other therapeutic modalities. What this means is that it has its own strengths and limitations. Some individuals benefit a lot but it fails in some circumstances. Knowing this fact helps us to be realistic when we use this strong tool.

To my understanding, the largest limitation of hypnosis is the fact that most hypnotic phenomena are temporary. That's why self-hypnosis and educating the subject are crucial to implementing and maintaining the treatment plan.

There are some ethical considerations of hypnosis to consider. Hypnosis should be used in an ethical manner and it should never be used as entertainment. As long as you use hypnosis as an honest persuasion art with the subject's consent and not as a deceptive trick, it's ethical.

You should also never use hypnosis for problems you are not qualified to deal with. This is particularly important when it comes to symptom therapy. You should never mask a symptom without understanding the underlying pathology.

Let's talk about the myths around hypnosis a little bit. Loss of control is the most common myth surrounding hypnosis. The truth is that even under the deepest trance states, the subject still has control over their thoughts and behaviors. For example, as a convincer technique, I may ask you to move if you can, and, surprisingly, you realize that you cannot move your body. Now, imagine that in this situation somebody yells, "Fire!" Suddenly you will jump up and the game will be over. In other words, you have voluntarily let go of control in hypnosis but you can take the lead whenever you decide to do so. Your observer mind keeps control of everything.

Having said that, in rare cases, there are conflicting findings suggesting that hypnosis can be abused by antisocial users. We have already discussed that briefly in ethical considerations.

Another myth about hypnosis is that you lose consciousness and have amnesia. The truth is that amnesia can happen only in deep hypnosis and in very few cases. Generally, the subject remembers everything after hypnosis.

The last thing to mention here is the importance of obtaining an informed consent form. Like any other treatment modality, you need to describe the limitations of the approach and explain the legalities simply.

CHAPTER 2

WHAT IS HYPNOSIS GOOD FOR?

In this chapter, we want to discuss the indications and applications of hypnosis. The medical indications will certainly be our priority.

Let's start with the most "exotic" indications for hypnosis in medicine. To illustrate, let me share with you the experience I had with an asthmatic patient. About eight years ago, I had a patient suffering from asthma. She had been on oral steroid medication for years. We had around five hypnosis sessions together. After that, her symptoms were well controlled without any steroids, at least for the six months I was doing follow up with her.

The other example is anesthesia. This application of hypnosis may look strange, for those who are not familiar with it. I'm not saying that it's cost effective or practical to apply hypnosis Instead of anesthesia in all cases. What I'm saying is that it can be applied in certain circumstances as an alternative.

In this chapter, I have just listed the indications with some very brief explanations about some of the conditions. Obviously, it's not possible to even name all the indications; but I hope this chapter helps you to have a general idea of some of the applications of hypnosis.

Please be informed that all the examples mentioned below are supported by clinical studies. You can find them easily in the medical literature, for example, through pubmed.com. Some of these clinical studies are randomized. Randomized clinical trials have the highest level of evidence in evidence-based medicine.

Hypnosis can be used in medical conditions like such as asthma, seasonal allergies, tinnitus, difficulty in swallowing pills, hiccups, rashes, and urinary retention.

It can be used for ego strengthening such as for enhancing esteem, confidence, and self-efficacy. It's also beneficial in anxiety disorders like phobias, panic attacks, and hypochondriasis which is also known as Illness Anxiety Disorder. In that condition, the patients strongly believe that they have a serious illness despite being physically well.

In cancer patients, hypnosis can be used for ego strengthening, self-healing and for controlling the side effects of chemotherapy.

Pain management is an important area when it comes to hypnotherapy including inflammation (like in arthritis), migraine headache, chronic pain, and fibromyalgia. Fibromyalgia is a syndrome affecting the soft tissue and is characterized by musculoskeletal pain.

Weight management is also among the most popular indications for hypnosis. It is useful for body image problems like body dysmorphic syndrome and anorexia nervosa or bulimia nervosa. Anorexia nervosa is characterized by needless and excessive weight loss. Bulimia nervosa is on the other end of the eating disorder spectrum and is characterized by extreme overeating followed by depression and self-induced vomiting.

Dissociative disorders are an important indication for hypnosis. There is a strong relationship between the risk of dissociative disorders and hypnotisability. On the other hand, highly hypnotizable patients with dissociative disorders respond much better to treatment. Common examples of dissociative disorders include PTSD or Post Traumatic Stress Disorder, Dissociative Identity Disorders or multiple personality and victims of sexual assault.

Insomnia and other sleep disturbances can also be helped by hypnosis. We should not forget the autoimmune disorders like lupus and scleroderma. Hypnosis is also very useful in habit disorders like nail biting. It is also widely used for smoking cessation.

Hypnodontics or hypnosis in dentistry is one of the most practical aspects of hypnosis. It can be used in cases of dental phobia, bruxism, TMJ dysfunction (a condition affecting muscles of the jaw), hypersensitive gag reflex and bleeding control.

Sports hypnosis uses hypnosis to help athletes enhance their performance. Studies show that hypnosis can enhance academic performances as well.

Hypnosis can also be used in sexual health. Sexual dysfunctions like premature ejaculation or psychologic impotence are some of the sexual indications for hypnosis.

Pediatrics is another important domain for hypnosis. We can manage a lot of abnormalities in children through hypnosis. For example, enuresis, stuttering, tics and more complicated forms of tics like Tourette's syndrome.

The benefits of hypnosis in the field of obstetrics and gynecology have also been studied in some clinical settings. Premenstrual syndrome is probably the most famous condition when it comes to hypnosis in gynecology. However, the indications of hypnosis in woman's health is not limited to that at all. For instance, hypnosis can help to ensure a comfortable delivery, it can help psychologic amenorrhea and hyperemesis gravidarum. (Hyperemesis gravidarum is severe nausea and vomiting as a complication of pregnancy.)

The important thing about the indications of hypnosis is the same as those for any other therapeutic modality. You need to approach the symptoms and condition wisely. There is no "one size fits all". For the sake of example, let's stick to smoking cessation. There is no magical solution with hypnosis when it comes to smoking but it is a powerful platform to execute your diagnostic and therapeutic approach. The 6-month abstinence rate after hypnosis is high enough though to consider hypnosis a reliable alternative to bupropion in smoking cessation. One of the simplest ways to approach a smoker is to induce nausea whenever he or she smokes. This can happen if the subject is hypnotizable enough. We will discuss that in the "Post Hypnotic Suggestions" as a hypnotic phenomenon later in this book in more detail. However, this approach is not the best one for two main reasons.

Firstly, it focuses on the symptoms and the presentation and the surface of the problem rather than the elimination of the underlying cause. Secondly, this effect is temporary and lasts -let's say- about half an hour.

The other approach is to use visualization techniques. For instance, under hypnosis, we may ask the subject to imagine the end results of smoking such as cancer, coronary artery disease or chronic obstructive pulmonary disease. This approach makes better sense but it's not the best in all cases.

Now let's assume we have found some footprints about the first smoking experience of the subject under hypnosis. It may happen when you try age regression with the patient. (We will talk more about age regression later in this book.) In this scenario, you may dive deeper using psychotherapy, cognitive therapy or N.L.P to modify the fundamental cognitions beneath- in the patient's subconscious mind.

The other approach is to use visualization in a positive way. Under hypnosis, the subject imagines healthy days without smoking. The subject repeats, "I used to be a smoker."

You may have noticed that hypnosis is not a therapy itself. On the other hand, it's a strong platform to execute the therapeutic approach. You induce the hypnosis and then use the proven "suggestion scripts" to approach the symptom. Please refer to the *Handbook of Hypnotic Suggestions and Metaphors* published by the American Society of Clinical Hypnosis to discover more about these scripts.

All said hypnosis is a therapy by itself in anxiety disorders.

The last thing I want to emphasize in this chapter is how to approach the problem in a holistic context when you are using hypnosis. Let's use an exaggerated example to dramatize the importance of the "context". Let's say you're trying to manage the self-esteem of a patient using hypnosis and it leads to a break up with his or her dominant partner. I'm not saying leave the dominant partner to exploit the power. What I'm saying is to approach the problem in a context and define a clear interactive objective with your client in advance.

CHAPTER 3

HOW TO INDUCE HYPNOSIS?

Well, this chapter is probably the most exciting one!

You are ready to learn the hypnosis induction techniques.

In this chapter, we discuss in brief how to induce hypnosis with the following techniques:

- Chiasson's technique
- Catalepsy
- Rapid eye roll induction
- Eye fixation
- Progressive relaxation
- Levitation
- Naturalistic
- Imagery technique
- Crasilneck's
- Eye opening & closing

Then we briefly discuss the hypnotisability tests.

Let's start with Chiasson's technique. To begin, you ask the subject to elevate his/her non-dominant hand and keep the hand above the eye line with the elbow bent. The reason for using the non-dominant hand is simply that it gets tired quickly. The reason behind keeping the hand above the eye line is to make gravity work in favor of your suggestion.

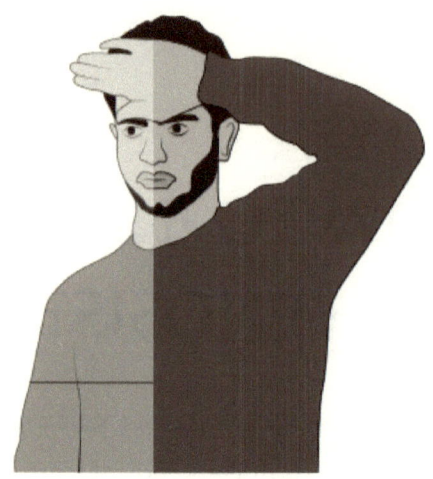

Now, I'll continue explaining the technique as if I'm speaking to the model: "Keep your fingers together. Just keep looking at the back of your hand. Your fingers start to spread, and your hand gets heavier and heavier. It looks like there is gravity between your eyes and your hand. Your hand is getting closer to your eye. Closer and closer … Heavier and heavier …"

The artistic part of the induction is to play with the tone of your voice to induce the trance smoothly.

"Not now but when your hand touches your face your eyelids will close if they are not already closed. You can close your eyes if you feel they are tired. You become deeply relaxed. Perfect. Your fingers are spreading more and more. Your hand is getting heavier and heavier and your hand is getting closer and closer to your face. I don't know which part of your hand touches your face. And to be honest, you don't know either. Just wait for your hand to touch your face. And when your hand touches your face, you go down to hypnosis."

You continue the suggestion with your own wording until the hand touches the face. When the subject's hand touches the face, you can say, "Your hand slowly comes down into your lap. And you go deeper and deeper."

Or you may say, "I may touch your hand, and help you to put your hand on the arm of your chair."

This provides you with the opportunity to combine Chiasson's technique with catalepsy as an induction technique. We'll talk more about catalepsy later in this book, either as an induction technique or a hypnotic phenomenon. You can also combine Chiasson's technique with other techniques like relaxation.

In practice, the hypnotherapist may combine or switch between different induction techniques based on the subject's feedback or the therapist's preference. Chiasson's is my favorite technique.

The second technique we discuss in this chapter is catalepsy. "Catalepsy is a nervous condition characterized by muscular rigidity"*

*Anticataleptic and antiepileptic activity of ethanolic extract of leaves of *Mucuna pruriens*: A study on role of dopaminergic system in epilepsy in albino rats

D. Champatisingh, P.K. Sahu, A. Pal, and G.S. Nanda

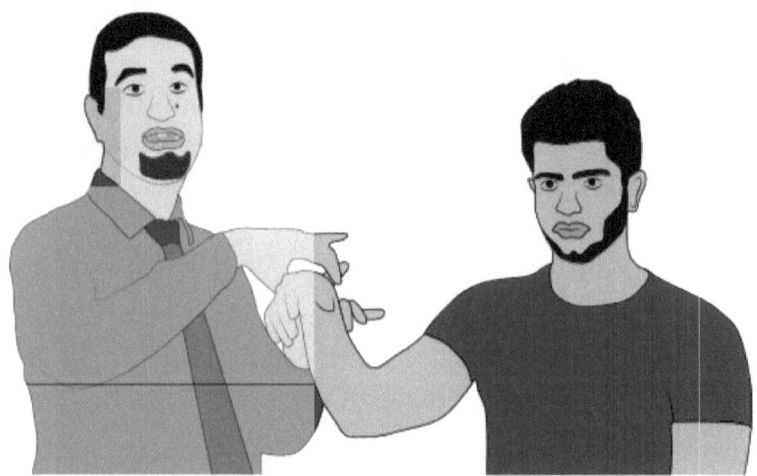

This rigidity can be associated with a loss of sensation. This makes catalepsy a phenomenon with the potential to be used in analgesia. Catalepsy is not only a hypnotic phenomenon, but it's also an induction or deepening technique. As an induction technique, catalepsy is started by creating confusion. The confusion element provides an opportunity for the subject to fixate their attention.

The best way is to hold the wrist from above. Then when the patient inhales, you remove the touch point. A very gentle movement, like you, are hanging the hand on a hook, facilitates the induction. You can keep touching different parts of the forearm with the other hand. You might conduct the "hanging maneuver" at the end of inhalation and beginning of exhalation.

Verbal suggestion can be used simultaneously with catalepsy. For instance, you can ask the subject to focus on their breathing or on the inhale or exhale. Keep making the distracting touches for a short while. You can leave the arm as it is but be careful not to leave it for too long. The subject may feel fatigue after or even during the hypnosis.

"Now, I slowly drop your hand on your lap."

You may continue catalepsy induction with hand levitation. If the subject is a new client, and you are still not familiar with the subject's hypnotic capacities, you can use a double bind suggestion like this:

"Your hand may develop a lightness and go up as if it's floating in the air or it may develop heaviness and go down on your lap."

Or

"I don't know if your hand gets heavier or lighter and which direction it goes."

As mentioned, catalepsy can also be used as a deepening technique after induction. Remember to let the subject know that you may touch his/her hand.

The next induction technique is rapid eye roll induction. This induction technique is suitable for emergency situations. It can induce hypnosis in less than a minute. You may combine catalepsy with "rapid eye roll" and measure the subject's pulse at the same time.

You ask the subject not to move their head and to follow your index finger. Then slowly move your fingers beyond the subject's visual field.

Or you may tell the subject:

"Roll your eyeballs up and slowly close your eyes."

I usually combine eye roll induction with an imaginary technique like this:

"Now imagine there is a gas in the air."

"Everybody can imagine like that."

"I don't know what color the gas is."

"And to be honest, you don't know either."

"But your unconscious mind knows exactly what color the gas is."

"What's the color that pops up in your mind?"

"Perfect."

"You are getting (for instance) the blue gas into your nose, airways, lungs, your blood circulation and all around your body and it makes you feel deeply relaxed and comfortable."

"Don't be in a rush."

"Take your time."

"Don't try to do anything."

"Just keep breathing and get the blue gas into your nose, airways and blood circulation."

"Perfect."

"Eye roll" is a good measure of hypnotisability as well. We'll discuss Spiegel's eye roll test later in this chapter.

Eye fixation is another induction technique. It is so simple. We ask the subject to stare at a point. The eyes get tired and then they close.

I'm not going to explain this technique in detail but, I will try to demonstrate the next technique, which is progressive relaxation. I combine that with an imagery technique:

"Imagine you are entering the water of a pool."

"You're using the poolside steps."

"The water temperature is perfect."

"You put your feet into the water."

"The waves of relaxation go up to your feet."

"Let the waves of relaxation expand to your ankles, legs, and knees."

"And you feel relaxed, deep and comfortable."

"Don't be in a rush."

"Take your time and enjoy."

"The waves of relaxation come into your thigh, front and back and make your muscles relax."

"And then your belt, abdomen, and back."

"The relaxation expands to your chest,"

"And the organs inside your chest."

"Including your heart and lungs."

"Let the waves come up to your shoulders,"

"And then arms, elbows, forearms, hands and fingers."

"And you feel relaxed, deep and comfortable."

"Don't be in a rush."

"Take your time and enjoy."

"The relaxation expands into your neck and the structures inside your neck."

"It goes up to your chin, mouth, lips, nose, cheeks."

"And your eyes."

"The waves expand to your forehead and your scalp."

"And even your hair."

Levitation is another induction technique that we are going to discuss in this chapter. Arm levitation is an advanced induction technique that was introduced by the great hypnotherapist, Milton Erickson.

This technique takes a long time. You can combine this technique with other techniques. However, it's not recommended to use progressive relaxation before arm levitation simply because the suggestions are opposite to each other.

You may use your touch to help the subject to levitate their hand. You may leave the hand cataleptic above or put it on the patient's lap. This technique works in three-quarters of all subjects.

You may switch the induction technique if you realize the subject is not responsive, despite the fact that you are spending time patiently.

When the subjects can be hypnotized by "arm levitation"; most probably they can also experience the "ideo-motor" phenomenon. We'll discuss the ideo-motor phenomenon later in this book in a separate chapter.

"Pay attention to your hands placed on your thighs."

"You can notice the feeling of your fingers."

"You may also have an idea in terms of the texture or temperature that your fingers are experiencing."

"Now, I want you to take a deep breath and watch how your hand becomes lighter."

"Normally, whenever you breathe in."

"Now watch how the feeling of texture changes when your hands become lighter."

"I don't know which hand starts to get lighter or which finger starts to go up."

"You may also notice very tiny movements on your fingers."

We don't discuss hand levitation in more detail here but feel free to study more about it. Each one of these techniques is actually a platform. So, you can add to them based on your creativity whenever you learn and practice the principles and feel comfortable then apply that in your practice. For instance, my preference is to add an imagery technique to arm levitation. I ask the subject to imagine a beautiful day in a local park.

"Lots of kids are playing with balloons in their hands."

"They leave their balloons and the balloons start to fly ..."

I think we've discussed the imagery techniques already. Naturalistic techniques are like imagery techniques. However, the context of imagination is more nature-oriented. Feel free to explore Crasilneck's technique on your own.

We'll explain about eye opening and closing in the next chapter when we talk about deepening techniques.

CHAPTER 4

HOW TO DEEPEN HYPNOSIS?

Let's start the deepening techniques with the description of the stages of trance. As mentioned earlier, moderate depth of hypnosis is enough for clinical purposes. Some perceptual changes are seen just in deep hypnosis, but these cognitive phenomena are not needed in most clinical settings. The best approach is to ask the patient to choose the depth of hypnosis that they would like. For instance, you may say:

"I don't know how deep you need to go for this session for the best results and, to be honest, you don't know either, but your subconscious mind knows exactly what depth is needed."

You may add an ideomotor technique to get feedback from the subject. We'll discuss the ideomotor phenomenon later in this book.

"Whenever you reach to the ideal depth level, your index finger that I'm touching now moves…"

Classically, the depths of hypnosis are categorized as light, medium and deep. Deep hypnosis is also called "somnambulistic". Some writers define a final stage called the stuporous stage. Having said that, there is no cut-off point between these stages. The phenomena experienced by the subject can be a benchmark for the depth of trance. A light trance is mostly associated with generalized relaxation. Catalepsy is usually observed in this stage. In a medium trance, different phenomena start to partially appear such anesthesia, amnesia and time distortion. The subject is still aware of the environment. In a deep trance, the hypnotic phenomena are presented in full. Some phenomena like hallucinations are only seen in a deep trance. The subject is highly suggestable when in deep hypnosis. In a deeper trance, the subject may experience depersonalization or loss of identity, loss of the concept of time and unitive experiences or feeling the potential to be anything or anyone.

There is no absolute distinction between the induction and deepening stages, and as a result of that, there's no cutoff point between induction and deepening techniques.

Let's start with the most powerful deepening technique, fractionation.

The whole concept of fractionation is to bring the subject in and out of a trance. This process deepens the hypnosis. With experience, you will realize that the more hypnosis sessions the subject has, the deeper the trance will be. Now, if you decrease the intervals between the sessions more and more, the deepening trend still exists. That's why you can even bring the subject in and out of a trance in one session, and it deepens the hypnosis.

You can wake the subject, keep the subject awake for one or two minutes, and then hypnotize him/her again. You can even decrease the intervals to five to ten seconds.

You can say:

"I count from one to three."

"You open your eyes."

"Look at my fingers and then close your eyes on my signal."

Another technique for fractionation is to keep the subject's eyes closed and say:

"Whenever I touch your right shoulder your hypnosis becomes deeper."

"Whenever I touch your left shoulder your trance gets lighter."

Then you can alternate between them, to deepen the depth. Another technique to leverage the depth of trance is to utilize the subject's motivation.

You may say:

"You go deeper and deeper because you want to (for instance) quit smoking."

In my experience, the subjects become deeper when they pay more and wait longer in the waiting room. Maybe I'm wrong and it's confirmation bias or maybe supply and demand works in the hypnosis world as well!

As discussed, most induction techniques can be used as deepening techniques. So, it's just a matter of spending time and being patient and expanding the induction creatively. Focusing on breathing always helps to deepen the trance. I usually add a kind of metaphor to that to deepen the hypnosis:

"Imagine there is a gas in the air."

"I don't know what color the gas is."

"And to be honest you don't know either."

"It can be green, blue, red, etc."

"By the way, what's the first color that pops up in your mind?"

Pause for a few seconds and evaluate the subject's facial expression and then continue:

"Perfect."

"You are breathing and getting the (for example) blue gas into your nose, airways, lungs, blood circulation and all around your body."

"And it makes you feel deep, relaxed and comfortable."

"Don't be in a rush."

"Just keep breathing and pay close attention to that."

"With each breath, you get more blue gas into your nose, airways, lungs and blood circulation."

"And it makes you deep, relaxed and comfortable."

See! Usually, there is no definite distinction between induction and deepening. Another effective deepening technique is using "downward movement metaphors". Some therapists prefer the staircase metaphor, but my personal preference is getting the subject to imagine an elevator going down.

You may start like this:

"You can imagine that you are in an elevator and the elevator is going down."

"Everyone can imagine like that."

"In each level, you take a deep breath and you become deeper and deeper."

And so on. When the subject gets to a desirable depth of hypnosis, it makes sense to save this depth level for the future by "anchoring". The anchoring means to associate a particular depth of hypnosis with a small ritual when the subject gets out of hypnosis. This ritual can be as simple as sitting in a particular chair in a particular place and breathing three times. I usually add a component of eye roll to the subject's ritual.

Like this:

"Now you are really deep."

"In future whenever you sit down on this chair in a quiet time and roll your eyes and close them"

"And take 3 deep breaths"

"You will experience this depth of trance."

Technically, using anchoring, in this case, is a post-hypnotic suggestion. We will talk more about post-hypnotic suggestions later on. Also, we'll dive deeper about that in the self-hypnosis chapter.

CHAPTER 5

HOW TO IMPLEMENT THE TREATMENT APPROACH?

As discussed earlier, the hypnotherapist should never use hypnosis for conditions that he or she is not qualified to deal with. This issue is more prominent because of the analgesic potentials of hypnosis. The inappropriate use of analgesia can mask the symptoms of a serious pathology.

Generally, hypnosis is a therapeutic modality. In some psychological contexts, it can be a diagnostic tool. The therapeutic nature of hypnosis magnifies the importance of making a clear diagnosis before applying hypnosis. In terms of diagnosis, the clinician should approach the symptoms through a classic differential diagnosis and exclude them one by one. This kind of diagnostic approach is beyond the scope of this book.

The assumption is that the readers of this book are qualified enough to make a precise diagnosis.

Now, let's focus on the therapeutic approach of hypnosis. Generally, there are five therapeutic approaches in hypnosis.

A-Imagination: for example, in ulcerative colitis, the subject may be asked to imagine what the distressed colon is like. Like a tunnel with red and inflamed walls. Highly hypnotizable subjects can be divided into two large categories- imaginative subjects who see pictures and colors and a dissociative group for whom the separation from the environment is more prominent. In the former category, the imagination can be a great platform to implement the treatment plan.

B-Metaphors: these are another form of imagination which can be indirectly used to implement the treatment approach. For instance, the patient with low self-esteem may imagine a strong tree. The metaphor is not necessarily in the form of imagination.

Past life therapy has been a source of controversy for years. In this book, we have a pragmatic view of that. In other word, if it helps us to manage the symptoms then why not to use it? We are not discussing the philosophical stuff here, and we are not about to prove or deny the reincarnation. All we need is to use it to treat the patients. You may assume that as a metaphor or a literal truth. I personally never suggest directly about past lives due to the risks of pseudo-memories. We will talk about pseudo-memories later in this book. However, if the patient tends to experience their past life in hypnosis, I don't resist that. I just keep going with the flow.

I once had an interesting experience in that regard. Years ago, I had an asthmatic patient who had been on oral steroid medication for years. During the hypnosis session, she mentioned that she had been hanged in what she called her previous life. After the hypnosis session, she came off the oral steroid medication and her symptoms were well managed by salbutamol spray only.

C-Suggestions: these are the backbone of the therapeutic approach. We implement the therapeutic approach through suggestions. Hypnosis is not a therapy by itself in most cases and an appropriate suggestion script should be used for treatment. The best thing to do is to use condition specific scripts that have been tested by other hypnotherapists in terms of efficiency during their years of practice.

I highly recommend the book *Suggestions and Metaphors* published by the American Society of Clinical Hypnosis. If you can't memorize the wording it's okay to read from the script. However, try to practice it again and again until you become comfortable enough to incorporate the script naturally into the hypnosis session.

D-Unconscious exploration: this is another therapeutic approach. In this case, hypnosis can be combined with cognitive therapy or psychotherapy. The age regression phenomenon provides an extra opportunity to dive into the unconscious mind and explore forgotten childhood experiences through hypnosis. We will discuss age regression further on in the book.

E- Hypnotic Phenomena. The last approach that we'll mention here is to use hypnotic phenomena for therapeutic purposes. The classic example is catalepsy. Because the cataleptic hand or foot does not feel pain or sometimes even touch, you can use catalepsy as an analgesic.

CHAPTER 6

HOW TO TERMINATE HYPNOSIS?

The termination part of hypnosis is usually neglected, and its importance is often underestimated. Without an appropriate termination, the trance will be unwrapped.

Let's continue this chapter by reviewing a myth about hypnosis:

"Some patients may stay in a trance state forever and never get out of it."

This is a complete myth. If you hypnotize a patient and leave them unattended, (which is not a good idea), two things may happen. The patient may fall asleep or they may become bored and open their eyes because of being left without any suggestion. The hypnosis will then be over.

In all the years I have been practicing hypnosis, I've just had one case of a subject who was difficult to rouse. I mistakenly hypnotized a patient with a histrionic personality disorder. I did not take enough time to obtain a good history and as a result of that, I missed the point that the patient had some histrionic traits. Even though there is no absolute contraindication to hypnotize patients with a personality disorder, it makes perfect sense not to do so.

We will discuss the indications and contraindications of hypnosis later. On that occasion, the patient was seeking attention through "becoming stuck in hypnosis". In other words, the patient was playing with me. However, that experience was more of a time wasting than a concerning situation.

An important thing to note about termination is that it's important to return all the temporary changes to the previous status before awakening the subject. Sometimes it can be clinically very significant. For example, in dentistry, a reasonable small amount of bleeding can prevent dry socket or alveolar osteitis. After the tooth extraction procedure, a clot is formed at the site to protect the alveolar bone beneath. That clot will facilitate wound healing. Too much bleeding can wash out the clot and increase the risk of dry socket. On the other hand, no bleeding, coagulation problems or too little bleeding, can cause failure to develop the clot properly and as a result of that, dry socket or alveolar osteitis occurs. If you stop bleeding during a dental procedure like tooth extraction using direct suggestions and forget to suggest to return it to as it was, you may potentially increase the risk of alveolar osteitis.

So, you need to reverse any suggestion you have made such as analgesia, muscle relaxation etcetera. The tone and volume of your voice should change gradually while leading the hypnosis towards the end.

The final suggestions will be about leaving the subject relaxed and happy for the rest of the day. My favorite way to terminate hypnosis is to count down:

"I'm going to count from ten to one and with each number, you'll feel more alert, awake and fresh. Nine is alert, eight is awake, seven is fresh and so on."

"At one you may open your eyes and come back to the room."

You can ask the subject to stay in hypnosis as long as he/she needs and then to awake. Sometimes this method is not practical due to time limitations.

It's important to ask the subject to stay in the waiting room for a while after hypnosis. They should not drive immediately.

When the subject is awakened you can see the sclera which is still congested. In this stage, if you ask the subject to close the eyes and get back to hypnosis, the patient will go into deep hypnosis again. It's called fractionation. We have already discussed fractionation in the deepening techniques.

At the end of hypnosis, you may ask if there are any comments or questions. I prefer to ask, "How was your experience?" Most of the time the patients smile and describe their experiences. It's a great opportunity for you to listen to them. The therapeutic session is not over yet. First, their feedback informs you about their hypnotisability. If they are highly hypnotizable, you may figure out what type of hypnotizable they are - imaginative or dissociative.

Rather than using the hypnotisability profile, you may get some information you were not able to get while the hypnosis was going on. For instance, the subject may give you some valuable information regarding what was experienced through age regression. This information can modify or direct your therapeutic approach to the problem.

CHAPTER 7

HYPNOTIC PHENOMENA

In this chapter, we try to define the most common hypnotic phenomena.

Let's start with catalepsy. **Catalepsy** is a neurological condition associated with muscular rigidity. Usually, the cataleptic limb does not feel any pain and that's why this phenomenon is important in hypnotic analgesia.

As discussed earlier, this phenomenon can be an induction technique, and a gateway for the subject to begin the trance. The interesting thing is that the cataleptic limb does not feel fatigue and pain.

You should consider asking the subject about conditions like arthritis, joint problems or vascular insufficiencies before hypnosis. A cataleptic hand is sensitive with these co-existing conditions because the limb loses two of the most important defense mechanisms, which are pain and fatigue.

Ideomotor activity is another hypnotic phenomenon. It's an involuntarily muscular reaction reflecting the subject's thoughts and feelings. The good news is that this phenomenon is common among patients. So, you can have an idea in terms of how and how fast the subject is following your suggestions.

Assume you are asking the subject to imagine an elevator is going down. You may say, "Whenever the elevator gets to the last level, your index finger that I'm touching now will move, and I'll see that you are on the last level.

There is overlap among catalepsy, ideomotor phenomenon, involuntarily hand movements and an inability to move. Some hypnotherapists assume that these phenomena are the same entity. To be on the safe side, we can at least assume that they belong to the same category.

Time distortion

The perception of time is almost always affected in hypnosis. Most of the time, the subject feels that the trance duration is shorter than it really is. This is called time contraction. In rare cases, when the subject's experience is not good in hypnosis, the duration of the session is perceived longer than it is. This is called time expansion. To verify whether your patient is experiencing time distortion or not, you may ask them, "Make a guess. How long do you think your hypnosis session lasted?" Most of the time when they look at their watches, they are surprised.

Amnesia:

Post-hypnotic amnesia is different from retrograde amnesia, which is a result of a brain injury or a psychological trauma in terms of reversibility. Post-hypnotic amnesia is temporary, and it can be conditioned or anchored to a simple cue. For example:

"When I touch your left shoulder, you will remember whatever you have forgotten."

Retrograde amnesia is not like that. It takes a lot of time and effort for a patient suffering from retrograde amnesia to remember what has been forgotten.

Post-hypnotic suggestion can be spontaneous or actively suggested. Clinically speaking, I think there is no point in suggesting amnesia actively. The good news is that hypnotic amnesia is safe and transient.

Pseudo memory is on the other end of the spectrum. Direct suggestions in deep hypnosis can create memories which do not really exist. One of the reasons I'm hesitant to suggest amnesia actively is because of the risk of creating pseudo-memories. Having said that, pseudo memory is not a concerning adverse effect and is self-limiting. The interesting thing about pseudo-memories is that sometimes the subject can distinguish between the pseudo-memories and the real ones, while sometimes the subject cannot differentiate between them.

Hypermnesia:

In some cases, the subjects can remember things easier under hypnosis. It does not mean that all those memories are accurate or reliable. Sometimes subjects can lie under hypnosis. The truth is that people can lie more easily under hypnosis because they become more imaginative. People can even believe in their own lies under hypnosis and those lies become the source of a pseudo-memory.

Hallucinations:

Hallucination can occur in two forms, positive and negative. Positive hallucinations mean seeing or sensing what does not exist. Negative hallucinations mean not seeing or sensing what really exists. Visual hallucinations are the hardest ones to experience and are seen in 3% of subjects.

Dissociation:

Dissociation is defined as separation, disconnection or detachment from the hypnosis room environment. As you know, this is the prominent feature of a special category of highly hypnotizable people. Sometimes you - as the therapist - lose communication with the patient experiencing dissociation and in some cases, the subject may present with automatic writing while experiencing dissociation. As a result of that, you can discover a lot in terms of what is going on behind the subject's mind and can explore their unconscious thought processes.

Dissociation can happen in conditions other than hypnosis too. Under extreme psychological or physical stresses, the mind uses dissociation as a defense mechanism. Actually, this mechanism is the underlying cause of PTSD or Post Traumatic Stress Disease.

Depersonalization:

When somebody gets disoriented, for example when a patient is experiencing delirium in a hospital, the sense of time is the first impaired sense. The patient cannot recognize what part of the day it is. If the patient becomes further disoriented, they also lose their sense of location. The patient cannot recognize and remember that they are at the hospital. In deeper disorientations, the patient cannot even remember their identity.

The same sequence is applicable to different depths of hypnosis. Almost all subjects experience some degree of time distortion. Some people in deeper hypnosis can experience dissociation. Some of them can experience depersonalization. In some cases, the subject can take on the identity of another person.

Unitive Experiences:

Maybe the extreme end of depersonalization is the unitive experience. Hypnosis is not the only way to experience unitive experiences but it's one of the ways. The subject feels the potential to be anybody or anything.

Out-of-Body Experience:

The extreme end of dissociation is an out-of-body experience. This phenomenon is reported in 3% to even 25% of the normal population, without even applying hypnosis. Some people experience it when they are in extremely stressful circumstances.

People can have an out-of-body experience in two major ways:

By experiencing the world as it is or by experiencing a fantasy world with huge distortions and deviations from conventional reality. Like meeting the wise, hookah-smoking caterpillar from the *Alice in Wonderland* story.

Somnambulism:

This is a deep trance experience with open eyes. There is a huge overlap between somnambulism and phenomena like dissociation.

Analgesia and Anesthesia:

The phenomena related to pain are among the most practical and useful ones. We know very little about how the underlying mechanism of it works though. We only can apply it in our daily practice.

However, it looks like the trance alternates the feeling of pain on a metacognition level. Metacognition is defined as a cognition (or insight) about another condition.

Let me give you an example. You have probably experienced that sometimes you don't remember the name of a famous actor whom you know very well. The name of the actor is a "cognition". The fact that you know that you know the actor is a "metacognition".

Back to pain relief in hypnosis. While the simple cognition of the pain still exists, the subject is unable to feel the sophisticated metacognitions, created "about" and on top of the simple cognitions. This theory (metacognition game) brings some controversies around the application of hypnosis in pain management. The same controversies have been around for analgesia and anesthesia as well.

In the operating theatre room, the anesthesiologist injects morphine to manage the intraoperative pain. Despite the fact that the patient is unconscious, he or she can still feel pain.

We can measure the SCEP or Somatosensory Cortical-Evoked Potentials, as an indicator of the pain felt by the patient unconsciously. So, if the morphine is not injected, tachycardia or hypertension may occur.

The same scenario is applicable to hypnosis. If the patient is not feeling pain, we should know that we are just blocking the output of the metacognition system. The patient is still feeling pain on another level. As a result of that, acute pain, particularly in invasive procedures, are not good indications for hypnosis. On the other hand, patients with chronic inflammatory pain are good candidates for hypnosis.

Some people are able to undergo major surgeries under hypnosis. Hypnosis plays the role of both an analgesic and anesthetic for them. Some people can experience analgesia to a lesser degree, or more in the affective component of pain rather than the sensory component. The bottom line is that more than 50% of people benefit from this phenomenon.

Hyperesthesia

The opposite of anesthesia is hyperesthesia. The affective component of pain is more enhanced in hyperesthesia. I have seen this phenomenon in PTSD patients.

Age Regression

Age regression means to relive a past event. It's much more than simply just remembering the past event. The voice, facial expression and even handwriting become childish. It's more of a perceptual change than a physiological one. Having said that, sometimes the changes look completely physiological.

The classic example of that is the Babinski sign. When the sole of the foot is stimulated by a blunt instrument, in normal adults, the involuntary response is downward flexion. The upward response or extension is called the Babinski sign. In normal adults, an upward response or a positive Babinski sign creates great suspicion of a serious illness like an upper motor neuron disease. In infants younger than 12 months, a positive Babinski sign is normal. The interesting part is that under hypnosis when you return the subject to the age of six months or earlier, their Babinski test becomes positive.

Age progression

Age progression is like imagining the future, however, the subject feels the experience in a more realistic way compared to just simple imagination.

Induced dreams

In some subjects, you can change the content of their dreams at night by suggestions.

CHAPTER 8

CAUTIONS, CONTRAINDICATION AND RESISTANCE

In this chapter, we will briefly discuss the contraindications for hypnosis.

There is no absolute contraindication for hypnosis. All the contraindications of hypnosis are relative.

Having said that, some therapists say that "stage" or "party hypnosis" is the only absolute contraindication.

We categorize contraindications of hypnosis into two large categories:

1-Pre-psychosis

2-Some personality disorders

Despite the fact that hypnosis never triggers a psychosis, it may reveal the symptoms in pre-psychosis. This may be interpreted as pushing a pre-psychotic patient into psychosis. To avoid all the controversies around that, it is recommended not to hypnotize a pre-psychotic patient.

1. **Pre-psychosis** is not difficult to diagnose if you invest enough time to interview the subject before the induction. A good history taking (including family history of psychosis) can clarify the situation.
2. **Personality disorders**. Let's start with the obsessive

personality disorder. It's very hard to hypnotize subjects with obsessive personality disorders. On the other hand, it's very easy to hypnotize people with histrionic personality disorders. Sometimes they want to show off, so, they pretend they are getting hypnotized. As a result of that, they really experience a deep trance. The issue is that they may do weird or unpredictable things. Sometimes, it's very hard to bring them out of hypnosis because they want to pretend that they are stuck in hypnosis and seek attention through that. Long story short, it makes sense not to hypnotize a subject with a histrionic personality disorder.

Borderline personality disorder is like histrionic personality disorder when it comes to hypnosis. As you may know, the prominent sign of borderline personality is splitting. In a simple definition, splitting is black and white thinking. They either love or hate someone or something. There is nothing in between. One of the complications you may see in those patients is transference and countertransference. However, transference and countertransference are not limited only to hypnosis or even to patients with personality disorders. It may occur during a normal counseling session with a normal client.

In transference, the subject unconsciously directs their emotions towards the therapist. In countertransference, the therapist makes such an unconscious emotional mistake toward the patient. It's like mistaking someone for someone else emotionally. Those adverse effects can be minimal and negligible, or extreme and affect the therapist-patient dynamic. They can disrupt the professional relationship completely. However, these extreme cases are very rare. They are seen in deep psychotherapy sessions and not during, for example, a simple hypnotic induction used for pain control.

In the paranoid cluster of personality disorders, it's almost impossible to induce hypnosis. Serious trust issues prevent you from conducting any effective intervention through hypnosis.

To wrap up, all the contraindications of hypnosis are relative and rare. Hypnosis is very safe to use, and you can apply it without any concern.

Now, let's review some adverse effects of hypnosis. These adverse effects are mild and almost always self-limiting. However, you need to know about them in order to educate your clients.

Signs of sympathetic overactivity like tachycardia and dry mouth are common in subjects experiencing hypnosis for the first time. They are rare among subjects who have already experienced hypnosis. Hypnosis is like a parasympathetic activity from the physiological point of view. As a result of that, the first time the body experiences hypnosis, through a structured hypnosis induction, it tries to compensate. As a rebound mechanism, sympathetic overactivity happens. This adverse effect is mild in nature and no intervention is necessary. You may just need to reassure the patient.

As mentioned earlier, pseudo-memories are another adverse effect. They can be erased as easily as they are created. To prevent pseudo-memories, avoid asking guiding questions and making direct suggestions. For instance, in deep hypnosis, don't ask, "Did you feel pain when you broke your leg in childhood?" If you do so, you may seed the memory of a broken leg or modify an existing memory in highly suggestable patients.

If a pseudo memory persists for a while, and the subject feels uncomfortable about that, you can hypnotize the subject again and remove that memory using appropriate reverse suggestions.

Stage Hypnosis and Party Hypnosis:

These are absolute contraindications of hypnosis. Adverse effects are reported commonly in these contexts.

Masking Physical Symptoms:

It's common sense not to mask pain or symptoms without diagnosing the underlying cause.

Liability Insurance:

Like any other practice, you need appropriate liability insurance coverage. Call your insurance agent and find out which insurers have experience with hypnotherapists.

Resistance:

Resistance to hypnosis can be voluntarily, involuntarily or a combination of both. It can be the result of miscommunication, wrong assumptions or beliefs in myths around hypnosis. Establishing a strong rapport and educating the patient resolve resistance most of the time.

Resistance management techniques are beyond the scope of this book. I will just mention a simple and quick technique here, which works in most cases.

The "Pretending" and "As if" technique:

When subjects are resisting consciously or unconsciously, or they think they are resisting, you may say:

"That's totally fine."

"It's pretty common."

"I just want you to pretend you are hypnotized."

You may show the client the manners and facial expressions of some hypnotized subjects. You may also ask them to pretend they have a cataleptic hand. Then in the second phase, ask them to role-play, as if even they cannot recognize themselves that they are hypnotized.

In the third attempt, make the induction as usual.

CHAPTER 9

SELF HYPNOSIS

It is important to inform the subject of the fact that every hypnosis is actually self-hypnosis. The role of the hypnotherapist is to be only a facilitator in the process.

The largest weakness of hypnosis is that the effects are temporary and need boosters. Those boosters are provided through self-hypnosis. Usually, the therapist teaches the subject how to hypnotize themselves after five or six sessions and designs a "weaning off" plan. Some subjects prefer to record the session and use it again as an alternative to self-hypnosis. I've never tried that, but a lot of my colleagues like this method.

Generally speaking, there are two methods of self-hypnosis.

The first method is to teach the subject to repeat a simplified version of induction or deepening script to themselves. This method does not always work effectively though.

A better alternative is to use anchoring. In other words, the therapist hypnotizes the subject and in deep hypnosis, conditions the subject to a stimulating behavior called anchoring. You can add a component of rapid eye induction to that anchoring. For example, in deep hypnosis, you may say, "Now you are in deep hypnosis. In the future, whenever you sit down on this chair in this quiet place and roll up your eyes and take three deep breaths, you will get to this depth of hypnosis."

"Don't be in a rush. Take your time and imagine you want to get back to this depth of trance. Everybody can imagine this. You sit down on this chair, take three deep breaths and get back to a deep trance. I won't talk for a while and will let you practice a few times until you feel quite comfortable with this exercise."

You need to prepare a tailored suggestion script, based on your treatment plan, and educate the patient in that regard. They can apply it when they want to induce self-hypnosis.

Patients' Compliance and Self Discipline

Years ago, I was under the impression that once you've taught self-hypnosis to a patient, your mission will have been accomplished.

I was wrong.

If the patient is not dedicated to continuing the therapeutic approach through self-hypnosis, not only the treatment result but also your professional performance and reputation will be in jeopardy. So, it's imperative to keep the client accountable somehow when it comes to daily self-hypnosis. For example, you may ask your receptionist to make some follow up calls.

If the patient is lacking the proper self-discipline, you need to postpone the self-hypnosis phase as much as possible. It means more sessions and more cost for the patient but sometimes that's the only way. When the patients see the results, there is a higher chance they will stay compliant. However, it's almost impossible to keep some patients dedicated enough. You need to explain that before starting the sessions and explain how important the patient's commitment to conduct the self-hypnosis is.

CHAPTER 10

CONVERSATIONAL HYPNOSIS

One of the definitions of hypnosis is found below:

"Hypnosis is the peak of rapport. The more we trust someone, the more we suspend our critical judgment and become more receptive to their suggestions."

Conversational hypnosis is very useful in some conditions.

For instance:
- Subjects who are resisting
- Anxiety management in dentistry
- Whenever you need to persuade the patient to make him or her compliant to the treatment

For sure, ethical considerations are very important. Honest persuasion can turn into deceptive tricks in the hands of an irresponsible therapist.

One of the famous covert or conversational techniques is a *truism*. Truism techniques are based on the assumption that the capacity for critical judgment will become desensitized if you repeat the obvious facts again and again. For example, imagine a security guard is checking everyone entering a dance club. If all the customers look legitimate and the security guard does not find anything unusual after checking, let's say, twenty guests, the guard will become desensitized and will not check the rest of them properly. Then the twenty-second person may bring a knife into the night club, and the security guard misses that. If the guest with a knife had been the first or second person, the security guard would never have missed that.

The mind works in the same way. The mind tends to generalize the facts, in order to simplify the analysis of overwhelming data coming from the environment. This generalization is learned through childhood development as a defense mechanism to cope with the huge amount of sensory signals coming to our mind at the same time.

You may start the conversation with the patient with emphasizing on an obvious fact. For example, the weather. If it's a beautiful sunny day, you may start by saying:

"It's a beautiful day and the sun is shining brightly."

You may continue describing the obvious conditions of the situation. Then at a certain time, you may use a linking statement like:

"As a result of that" and then make your suggestion:

"I will be your candidate of choice!"

It's not important that there is no logical relation between the truth in the first statement and the suggestion. Even if the subject realizes that this reasoning is illogical, they will be still receptive to the suggestion.

It is important not to use "but" as a linking statement as this word sharpens the critical judgment momentarily. The best linking statement in this context is simply "and".

Pacing and leading:

The "pacing and leading" technique is pretty much the same. You start the process by mirroring the subject's body language. Let me give you an example. Imagine that you are a dental assistant and a patient with dental phobia comes over to your office for an appointment. You may mirror not only the patient's body language but also their facial expression. You may smile and be welcoming and still mirror the patient's anxiety till you realize that the synchronization has happened.

Then you will lead the situation. The best way to lead the situation is by breathing deeply and watching how the patient follows you. Breathing is my favorite technique for three purposes:

1-As the pacing technique: I try to mirror the patient's breathing pattern as much as I can.

2-As the leading technique: to make the patient relaxed through deep breaths when I realize the patient is following me.

3-As a litmus test to see if the synchronization has happened or not.

You may be creative and use your own ways to apply these principles. Pacing and leading and other conversational techniques take a lot of practice to be master and are very artistic. You need to apply, fail, modify and optimize the technique to feel quite confident about using that in your daily practice. It's like learning how to play the guitar.

The mirroring phase may not be necessarily through body language.

You may even mirror the patient's emotions or even agree with their ideas as the pacing phase.

We will create a separate course about conversational hypnosis in the future. In this chapter, I just wanted to share with you the basics in that regard.

CHAPTER 11

HOW TO EDUCATE YOUR CLIENTS?

I've added this chapter realizing that a lot of practitioners are concerned about their clients' perception about hypnosis. Before that, I was merely focusing on health care professionals' perception of hypnosis.

The objective of this chapter is to discuss briefly how to educate your clients about hypnosis and help them to have a realistic perception of the process in a short period of time.

Maybe the most effective icebreaker to open the conversation is to mention some of the myths surrounding hypnosis. We have already discussed a few of those myths. Unfortunately, the first impression of a naïve client about hypnosis has mostly been created either by a stage hypnotist in a recreational context or by a Hollywood movie. Neither of them is a realistic illustration of the objectives in hypnotherapy.

Discussing the myths around hypnosis is like a gate opener into your client's concerns. Based on my experience, when you address the myths around hypnosis, and answer the client's questions, within a short period of time, like twenty minutes or so, you are able to provide an overview of what they are going to experience. You'll then be able to set their expectations.

You can discern the patients who have magical or supernatural perceptions of hypnosis very quickly. Then you can make mention of those subjects. They then have two options:

1-To align their perception about hypnosis with yours

2- Forget about hypnosis as a therapeutic modality.

It's very important to be assertive at this point and tell the subject frankly if they have been misled by a Hollywood movie or something else. Hypnosis is a process about their health and they need to be realistic about that. If your subject is educated about medical topics and psychology, feel free to explain what you do and why you do certain things even during the hypnosis session while the subject is under hypnosis.

When I started practicing hypnosis, I was concerned that if I discussed the process and technicalities with the patient while they were in a trance, it might distract them from the therapy plan or affect the depth of hypnosis. After a while, I realized that it's exactly the opposite.

If the subject is familiar with related terminology and interested in discussing the details, feel free to share the information about the procedure and the rationale behind each step as much as possible. Otherwise, If they are just looking for the result and are not interested in the technicalities, then it does not make sense to bother them with what is interesting to you (and me!) and not necessarily to them.

Another important thing to mention is the possible adverse effects. Reassure them that if any, they would be mild and self-limiting. As mentioned earlier, patients who are undergoing hypnosis for the first time may experience the symptoms of sympathetic overactivity such as heart palpitations. When the patient knows that this is mild and self-limiting, he or she will be able to handle that easily. It is important particularly when the primary issue is anxiety or anxiety related.

The key to success in hypnotherapy is to keep the channel of communication open as much as possible during all stages of treatment. It's never like prescribing medication and just moving on. You need to interact with the patient and experience the therapy yourself in each individual step.

CHAPTER 12

HYPNOSIS FOR COMPASSION FATIGUE

In the previous chapter, we mentioned that the hypnotherapist should be actively involved in their patients' treatment. This may affect the therapist's objectivity to some extent, and as a result of that, the therapist may absorb some of the negative experiences over time. This is called "compassionate fatigue" and is seen in all healthcare professionals and even in lawyers. It's more serious in professionals dealing with traumatized or sexually abused patients.

It this short chapter, I want to emphasize that hypnosis is a strong tool for healthcare professionals to manage their own "compassionate fatigue" which is also known as "secondary traumatic stress" or "STS". Daily self-hypnosis is a great tool for the therapist to use to overcome STS in the long term.

My favorite metaphor for the therapists' STS is "taking a shower". You may imagine, for example at the end of the day before taking an actual shower, that you are taking a shower and washing away all the negative experiences that you've been exposed to through your clients. You're washing them down the shower drain.

If you face some persistent negative pictures, don't resist. Just pause with washing them out. Keep them and apply some simple N.L.P or neurolinguistic programming techniques to them. For example, watch how your feelings change when you make the picture smaller or larger or you change the colors. Your feelings will become weaker when you play with the pictures. Then you may get back to the metaphor and wash out the annoying experiences.

All this might happen during a daily self-hypnosis session. At the time of writing this book, I'm working with a group of caregivers to help them manage their daily stresses. Some of them are non-professional caregivers helping family members.

Feel free to contact me and share your experiences when you use hypnosis to help such clients.

www.ingramcontent.com/pod-product-compliance
Lightning Source LLC
Chambersburg PA
CBHW030019190526
45157CB00016B/3135